30-Minute Cancer-Fighting Recipes

Harness the Healing Power of Your Body with Quick Recipes for Optimal Health

Dr. Olivia Paul

This Book belongs to:

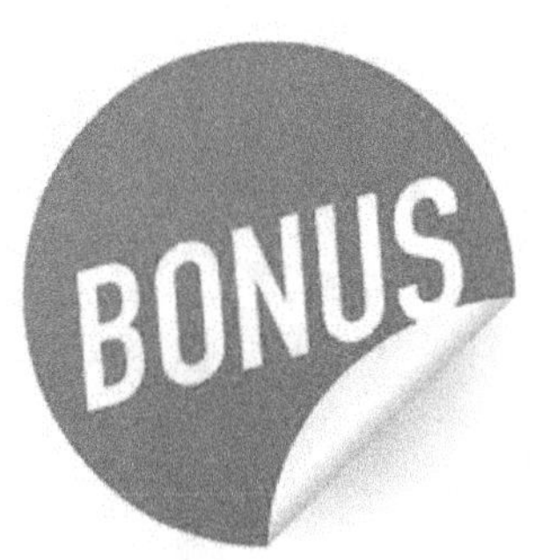

30-DAY

MEAL

PLANNER

TABLE OF CONTENTS

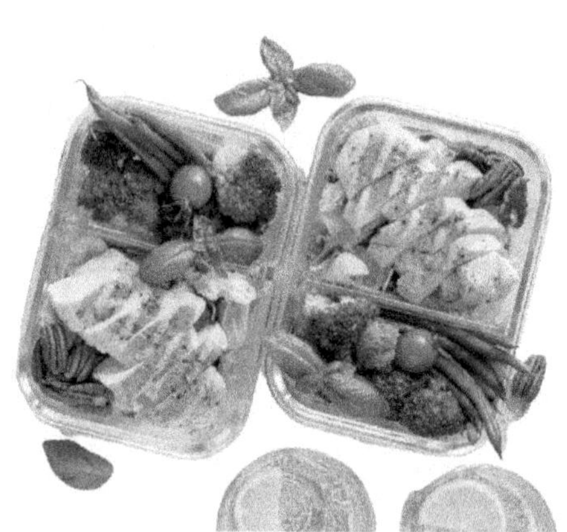

Introduction

Welcome to "30-Minute Cancer-Fighting Recipes," a collection of quick and delicious recipes designed to nourish your body, support your health, and empower you in your journey against cancer. In this book, we will explore the incredible power of food and its potential to fight cancer and promote overall well-being.

Each recipe in this collection has been carefully crafted with cancer-fighting ingredients, packed with antioxidants, and designed to provide you with the essential nutrients your body needs. But this book is not just about food; it is about embracing a lifestyle that promotes health and healing.

In my own personal journey, I witnessed the transformative impact of making conscious choices in my diet and lifestyle. I saw how a nourishing meal could bring comfort, strength, and a renewed sense of hope. It was through experimenting with different ingredients, flavors, and cooking techniques that I discovered the immense potential of food as medicine.

This book is a culmination of my experiences, research, and passion for creating meals that are not only delicious but also support your body's natural defenses against cancer. I invite you to join me on this journey, to unlock the healing power of food, and to nourish yourself in ways that promote vitality, resilience, and well-being. Together, let us thrive in health and fight cancer one delicious recipe at a time.

Chapter 1: Understanding Cancer-Fighting Ingredients

The Power of Antioxidants

In the fight against cancer, it is crucial to arm our bodies with powerful weapons that can help protect against oxidative stress and cellular damage. One such weapon in our arsenal is the power of antioxidants. These incredible compounds found in various foods can play a pivotal role in supporting our overall health and well-being. In this chapter, we will delve into the world of antioxidants and their profound impact on cancer prevention and management. We will explore their mechanisms of action, their role in reducing inflammation and oxidative stress, and their ability to support our immune system.

Understanding Antioxidants:

Antioxidants are substances that can inhibit or neutralize free radicals, which are unstable molecules that can cause cellular damage and contribute to the development of various diseases, including cancer. They work by donating an electron to stabilize the free radicals, preventing them from causing further harm to our cells.

Types of Antioxidants:

There are several types of antioxidants, each with its unique properties and health benefits. Some well-known antioxidants include vitamin C, vitamin E, beta-carotene, selenium, and flavonoids. These antioxidants can be found in a wide range of fruits, vegetables, nuts, seeds, and whole grains.

Benefits of Antioxidants in Cancer Prevention:

Numerous studies have demonstrated the potential of antioxidants in reducing the risk of cancer and supporting cancer treatment. They can help neutralize harmful free radicals, inhibit the growth of cancer cells, protect DNA from damage, and support the body's natural detoxification processes. Antioxidants also play a crucial role in reducing inflammation, which is a hallmark of many chronic diseases, including cancer.

Top Antioxidant-Rich Foods:

Including antioxidant-rich foods in our daily diet is essential for harnessing their protective effects. Some of the top antioxidant-rich foods include berries, dark leafy greens, cruciferous vegetables, citrus fruits, nuts, seeds, and spices like turmeric and cinnamon. Incorporating these foods into our 30-minute cancer-fighting recipes can amplify their health benefits and enhance the flavor and nutritional profile of our meals.

Cooking Techniques to Preserve Antioxidants:

While antioxidants are highly beneficial, they can be sensitive to heat and light. Therefore, it is important to adopt cooking techniques that help preserve their potency. Methods like steaming, sautéing, and stir-frying can help retain the antioxidant content in our ingredients. Avoiding prolonged cooking times and excessive heat exposure can also help maintain the nutritional integrity of our meals.

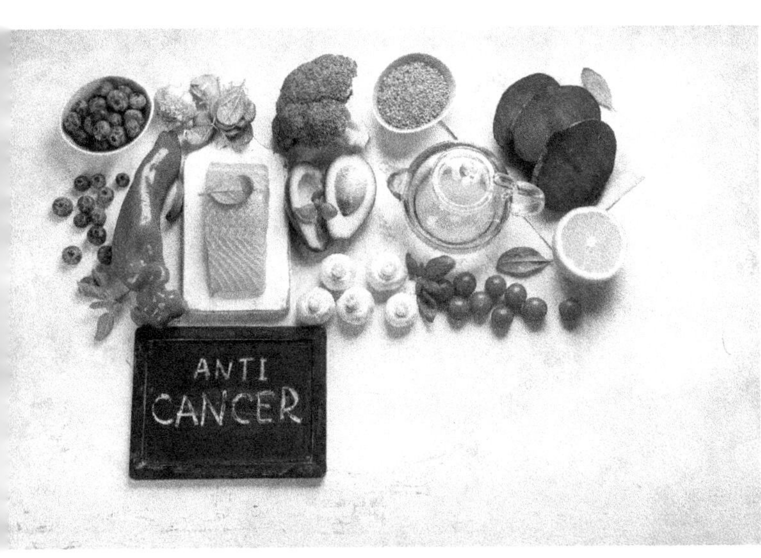

Creating Antioxidant-Rich 30-Minute Recipes:

Now that we understand the power of antioxidants, it's time to put this knowledge into action. In the following chapters, you will find a collection of 30-minute cancer-fighting recipes that are not only delicious but also packed with antioxidant-rich ingredients. From vibrant salads to hearty stews and energizing smoothies, these recipes have been carefully curated to provide you with a diverse range of flavors and nutrients to support your health and well-being.

Conclusion:

The power of antioxidants in our fight against cancer cannot be overstated. By incorporating antioxidant-rich foods into our daily diet and preparing them through gentle cooking methods, we can harness their full potential and enjoy their incredible health benefits. As we embark on this journey of 30-minute cancer-fighting recipes, let us remember the profound impact that antioxidants can have on our overall well-being. Together, let us embrace the power of antioxidants and nourish our bodies to thrive in health and vitality.

Superfoods for Cancer Prevention

In the fight against cancer, prevention is key. While there is no magical food that can guarantee protection against this complex disease, research has shown that certain foods, known as superfoods, possess exceptional nutritional properties that may help reduce the risk of cancer. Superfoods are packed with vitamins, minerals, antioxidants, and phytochemicals, making them potent allies in promoting overall health and well-being. In this article, we will delve into the world of superfoods for cancer prevention, exploring their unique qualities, the scientific evidence supporting their benefits, and how to incorporate them into a balanced and nutritious diet.

Understanding Superfoods:

Superfoods are nutrient-dense foods that offer a myriad of health benefits due to their rich concentrations of essential nutrients and bioactive compounds. They are often rich in antioxidants, which are powerful substances that help neutralize harmful free radicals in the body, reducing oxidative stress and protecting against cellular damage. Additionally, superfoods may have anti-inflammatory properties and contain phytochemicals that have been shown to exhibit anti-cancer effects.

Superfoods for Cancer Prevention:

Numerous superfoods have been identified for their potential in cancer prevention. These include berries, cruciferous vegetables, leafy greens, turmeric, garlic, green tea, mushrooms, flaxseeds, and many more. Each superfood possesses its own unique combination of nutrients and bioactive compounds that contribute to its cancer-fighting properties. For example, berries are rich in antioxidants and fiber, which can help reduce inflammation and oxidative stress. Cruciferous vegetables, such as broccoli and kale, contain sulforaphane and indole-3-carbinol, compounds known for their potential to inhibit cancer cell growth and promote detoxification processes in the body.

Scientific Evidence and Cancer Prevention:

Numerous studies have explored the relationship between superfoods and cancer prevention, yielding promising results. For instance, research suggests that the antioxidants found in berries may help protect against various types of cancer, including breast, colon, and prostate cancer. The bioactive compounds in cruciferous vegetables have been shown to possess anti-cancer properties, particularly in relation to lung, colorectal, and breast cancer. Turmeric, a spice widely used in Indian cuisine, contains curcumin, which has demonstrated anti-inflammatory and anti-cancer effects in laboratory studies. Green tea, another notable superfood, is rich in catechins, which have been associated with a lower risk of several cancers, such as breast, prostate, and colorectal cancer.

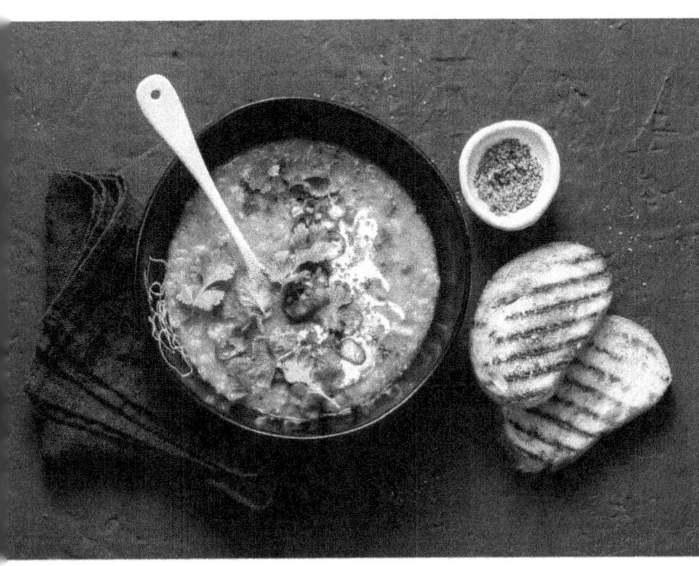

Incorporating Superfoods into a Cancer-Fighting Diet:

Integrating superfoods into your daily diet doesn't have to be complicated. There are countless creative and delicious ways to enjoy these nutrient powerhouses. Start by incorporating a variety of superfoods into your meals and snacks. For example, add berries to your breakfast yogurt or oatmeal, include a generous serving of leafy greens in your lunchtime salad, incorporate turmeric into your curry dishes, and snack on a handful of nuts and seeds for a dose of healthy fats and essential nutrients. Additionally, experiment with different cooking methods, such as steaming or lightly sautéing vegetables, to preserve their nutritional content.

Creating Balanced and Nutritious Meals:

While superfoods play a crucial role in cancer prevention, it's important to remember that a holistic approach to nutrition is essential. Focus on creating a well-rounded and balanced diet that includes a variety of fruits, vegetables, whole grains, lean proteins, and healthy fats. Avoid relying solely on superfoods and instead aim for a diverse array of nutrient-dense ingredients. By incorporating a wide range of foods, you can ensure that you're obtaining all the necessary nutrients for optimal health and well-being.

The Importance of a Healthy Lifestyle:

While superfoods offer significant benefits, it's important to remember that they are just one piece of the puzzle when it comes to cancer prevention. A healthy lifestyle encompasses more than just diet. Engaging in regular physical activity, managing stress levels, maintaining a healthy weight, avoiding tobacco and excessive alcohol consumption, and practicing sun safety are all crucial factors in reducing cancer risk. When combined with a nutrient-rich diet that includes superfoods, these lifestyle choices can have a powerful impact on overall health and well-being.

Lastly:

Superfoods for cancer prevention are a valuable addition to a healthy and balanced diet. The wide array of nutrients and bioactive compounds found in these foods can help protect against cellular damage, reduce inflammation, and support the body's natural defense mechanisms. However, it's important to approach cancer prevention holistically, incorporating a variety of healthy lifestyle choices alongside a nutrient-rich diet. By harnessing the power of superfoods and adopting a comprehensive approach to well-being, you can take proactive steps towards reducing your risk of cancer and promoting long-term health.

The Importance of Phytochemicals

Phytochemicals, also known as phytonutrients, are natural compounds found in plants that are responsible for their vibrant colors, flavors, and aromas. While phytochemicals are not considered essential nutrients like vitamins and minerals, they offer numerous health benefits and play a crucial role in supporting overall well-being. These bioactive compounds have been extensively studied for their potential to prevent chronic diseases, including cancer, heart disease, diabetes, and neurodegenerative disorders. In this article, we will explore the importance of phytochemicals in maintaining optimal health, understand their diverse functions, and discover how to incorporate them into a balanced diet.

The Diverse World of Phytochemicals:

Phytochemicals are incredibly diverse, with thousands of different compounds identified to date. Some well-known examples include flavonoids, carotenoids, phenolic acids, glucosinolates, and curcuminoids. Each class of phytochemicals possesses unique properties and functions, contributing to their health-promoting effects. For instance, flavonoids are powerful antioxidants that help protect cells from damage caused by free radicals, while carotenoids provide the vibrant colors in fruits and vegetables and have been linked to eye health and cancer prevention. Phenolic acids, found in foods such as berries and coffee, have anti-inflammatory and antioxidant properties that support cardiovascular health.

The Health Benefits of Phytochemicals:

Phytochemicals offer a wide range of health benefits, primarily due to their antioxidant and anti-inflammatory properties. These compounds work together to combat oxidative stress, reduce chronic inflammation, and protect against cellular damage. By neutralizing harmful free radicals, phytochemicals help prevent DNA damage and promote healthy cell function. Research suggests that phytochemical-rich diets are associated with a lower risk of chronic diseases, including cancer, cardiovascular disease, diabetes, and age-related macular degeneration. Additionally, phytochemicals may support immune function, improve cognitive health, and promote healthy aging.

Phytochemicals and Cancer Prevention:

One area where the importance of phytochemicals shines is in cancer prevention. Many phytochemicals have demonstrated powerful anti-cancer effects, including inhibiting the growth of cancer cells, inducing programmed cell death (apoptosis), and suppressing tumor formation. For example, the compound curcumin, found in turmeric, has been extensively studied for its anti-inflammatory and anti-cancer properties. Resveratrol, found in grapes and red wine, has shown promise in preventing the development and progression of various cancers. Sulforaphane, abundant in cruciferous vegetables like broccoli and cauliflower, has been linked to reduced cancer risk, particularly in breast, prostate, and colorectal cancers.

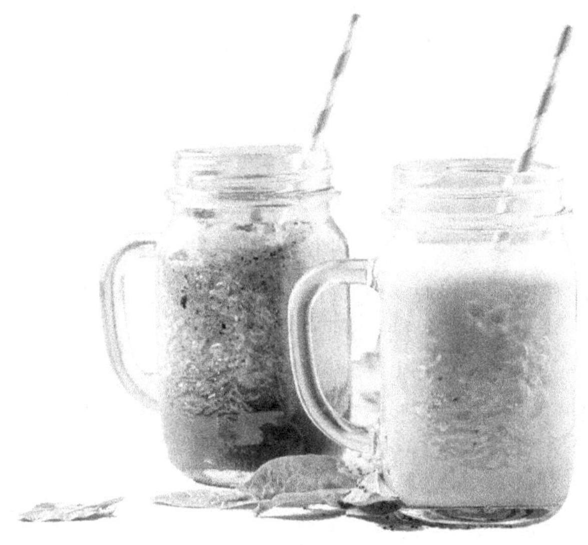

Incorporating Phytochemicals into a Balanced Diet:

The key to reaping the benefits of phytochemicals lies in consuming a diverse array of plant-based foods. Fruits, vegetables, whole grains, legumes, herbs, and spices are all rich sources of phytochemicals. To maximize their intake, aim for a colorful plate filled with a variety of produce. Include berries, citrus fruits, leafy greens, cruciferous vegetables, tomatoes, peppers, and whole grains in your meals and snacks. Additionally, incorporate herbs and spices like turmeric, ginger, garlic, and cinnamon to enhance flavor and boost phytochemical content. Opting for organic and locally sourced produce can also ensure higher nutrient density and minimize exposure to pesticides.

Synergistic Effects of Whole Foods:

While it's tempting to rely solely on supplements or isolated phytochemical extracts, research suggests that the greatest health benefits come from consuming whole foods. Whole foods contain a complex mixture of phytochemicals that work synergistically to enhance their bioavailability and effectiveness. The intricate interactions between different compounds within a food matrix contribute to their overall health-promoting effects. Therefore, prioritize whole, minimally processed foods over supplements whenever possible.

Incorporating Phytochemicals into Everyday Recipes:

Adding phytochemical-rich foods to your daily meals is easier than you might think. Start by incorporating a variety of fruits and vegetables into your salads, smoothies, and stir-fries. Experiment with different herbs and spices to enhance the flavor and nutritional content of your dishes. For example, sprinkle turmeric and black pepper into your scrambled eggs or roasted vegetables. Blend berries and leafy greens into a nutritious smoothie. Incorporate legumes like lentils, chickpeas, and black beans into soups, stews, and salads. By getting creative in the kitchen, you can enjoy delicious meals while reaping the benefits of phytochemicals.

Conclusion:

Phytochemicals are nature's powerful allies in promoting optimal health and preventing chronic diseases, including cancer. These bioactive compounds found in plant-based foods offer a wide array of health benefits, from reducing inflammation and oxidative stress to inhibiting tumor growth and supporting immune function. By incorporating a diverse range of phytochemical-rich foods into your diet, you can harness their potential and support your overall well-being. Remember, a balanced and varied approach to nutrition, along with other healthy lifestyle choices, is key to reaping the full benefits of phytochemicals and reducing the risk of chronic diseases. Embrace the power of phytochemicals and nourish your body with the vibrant flavors and healthful benefits of plant-based foods.

Chapter 2: Breakfast and Brunch Recipes

Energizing Green Smoothie

Ingredients:

- ✓ 1 ripe banana
- ✓ 1 cup spinach leaves
- ✓ 1 cup kale leaves
- ✓ 1/2 cucumber, peeled and chopped
- ✓ 1/2 green apple, cored and chopped
- ✓ 1 tablespoon chia seeds
- ✓ 1 tablespoon almond butter
- ✓ 1 cup unsweetened almond milk or coconut water
- ✓ Ice cubes (optional)

Instructions:

1. Peel the banana and chop it into chunks.
2. Rinse the spinach and kale leaves thoroughly.
3. In a blender, combine the banana, spinach, kale, cucumber, green apple, chia seeds, almond butter, and almond milk or coconut water.
4. Blend on high speed until all the ingredients are well combined and the mixture is smooth.
5. If desired, add ice cubes to the blender and blend for a few more seconds to make the smoothie chilled.
6. Pour the smoothie into glasses and serve immediately.
7. You can garnish the smoothie with additional chia seeds or a slice of green apple, if desired.

Note: Feel free to adjust the quantities of ingredients based on your taste preferences. You can also add a squeeze of lemon juice or a handful of fresh mint leaves for added freshness and flavor. Enjoy this energizing green smoothie as a refreshing and nutritious start to your day or as a healthy snack any time.

Quinoa Breakfast Bowl

Ingredients:

- ✓ 1 cup cooked quinoa
- ✓ 1/2 cup almond milk or any milk of your choice
- ✓ 1 tablespoon honey or maple syrup
- ✓ 1/2 teaspoon vanilla extract
- ✓ 1/4 cup sliced fresh fruits (such as berries, banana, or kiwi)
- ✓ 2 tablespoons chopped nuts (such as almonds, walnuts, or pecans)
- ✓ 1 tablespoon chia seeds
- ✓ 1 tablespoon shredded coconut (optional)

Instructions:

1. In a saucepan, heat the cooked quinoa with almond milk over medium heat. Stir occasionally until the mixture is warm and creamy.
2. Stir in honey or maple syrup and vanilla extract, and continue to cook for another minute or until well combined.
3. Remove the quinoa mixture from heat and transfer it to a bowl.
4. Top the quinoa with sliced fresh fruits, chopped nuts, chia seeds, and shredded coconut, if desired.
5. Mix all the ingredients together gently to ensure they are evenly distributed.
6. Serve the quinoa breakfast bowl warm or chilled, according to your preference.
7. Note: Feel free to customize your quinoa breakfast bowl with your favorite toppings such as dried fruits, seeds, or a drizzle of nut butter. You can also add a sprinkle of cinnamon or a dash of cocoa powder for extra flavor. This nutritious and filling breakfast bowl is a great way to start your day with a boost of energy and essential nutrients from quinoa and fresh fruits.

Avocado Toast with Smoked Salmon

Ingredients:

- ✓ 2 slices of whole grain bread
- ✓ 1 ripe avocado
- ✓ 4 ounces smoked salmon
- ✓ 1 tablespoon fresh lemon juice
- ✓ Salt and pepper to taste
- ✓ Optional toppings: sliced tomatoes, red onion, capers, or microgreens

Instructions:

1. Toast the slices of whole grain bread until they are golden and crispy.
2. While the bread is toasting, cut the avocado in half and remove the pit. Scoop the avocado flesh into a bowl and mash it with a fork until smooth.
3. Add the fresh lemon juice to the mashed avocado and season with salt and pepper to taste. Mix well.
4. Spread the mashed avocado mixture evenly onto the toasted bread slices.
5. Top the avocado toast with smoked salmon, arranging it in an even layer.
6. If desired, add additional toppings such as sliced tomatoes, red onion, capers, or microgreens for extra flavor and texture.
7. Serve the avocado toast with smoked salmon immediately and enjoy!

Note: Avocado toast with smoked salmon is a delicious and nutritious option for breakfast, brunch, or a light meal. The creamy avocado pairs perfectly with the smoky flavor of the salmon, creating a satisfying and flavorful combination. Feel free to customize your avocado toast by adding your favorite ingredients or experimenting with different toppings.

erry Chia Pudding

gredients:

- ✓ 1/4 cup chia seeds
- ✓ 1 cup almond milk (or any milk of your choice)
- ✓ 1 tablespoon maple syrup or honey
- ✓ 1/2 teaspoon vanilla extract
- ✓ 1 cup mixed berries (such as strawberries, blueberries, raspberries)
- ✓ Optional toppings: additional berries, shredded coconut, chopped nuts

structions:

1. In a bowl, combine the chia seeds, almond milk, maple syrup or honey, and vanilla extract. Stir well to make sure the chia seeds are evenly distributed. Let the mixture sit for 5 minutes.

2. After 5 minutes, stir the chia seed mixture again to break up any clumps that may have formed. Place the bowl in the refrigerator and let it sit for at least 2 hours or overnight to allow the chia seeds to absorb the liquid and create a pudding-like consistency.

3. Once the chia pudding has thickened, give it a good stir to make sure it is well combined.

4. In a separate bowl, mash or blend half of the mixed berries to create a berry sauce. You can leave some berries whole for added texture.

5. To assemble the pudding, layer the chia pudding and the berry sauce in serving glasses or bowls. Start with a layer of chia pudding, followed by a layer of berry sauce, and repeat until all the pudding and sauce is used.

6. Top the pudding with additional berries, shredded coconut, or chopped nuts for added flavor and texture, if desired.

7. Serve the berry chia pudding chilled and enjoy as a healthy and satisfying breakfast, snack, or dessert!

Note: Berry chia pudding is a nutrient-rich and delicious treat packed with antioxidants and omega-3 fatty acids from the chia seeds, and vitamins and minerals from the mixed berries. The natural sweetness of the berries pairs perfectly with the creamy texture of the chia pudding. Feel free to customize your berry chia pudding by using your favorite berries and adding your preferred toppings. Enjoy this nutritious and flavorful pudding as a part of your balanced and healthy diet.

Chapter 3: Lunch and Dinner Recipes

Grilled Salmon with Lemon and Dill

Ingredients:

- ✓ 2 salmon fillets (6-8 ounces each)
- ✓ 2 tablespoons fresh lemon juice
- ✓ 2 tablespoons olive oil
- ✓ 2 cloves garlic, minced
- ✓ 1 tablespoon fresh dill, chopped
- ✓ Salt and pepper, to taste
- ✓ Lemon wedges, for serving

Instructions:

1. Preheat the grill to medium-high heat.
2. In a small bowl, whisk together the lemon juice, olive oil, minced garlic, chopped dill, salt, and pepper.
3. Place the salmon fillets on a plate or in a shallow dish and pour the marinade over them, making sure they are well coated. Let the salmon marinate for about 15-20 minutes to allow the flavors to infuse.
4. Once the grill is hot, lightly oil the grates to prevent the salmon from sticking. Place the salmon fillets on the grill, skin-side down.
5. Close the grill and cook the salmon for about 4-6 minutes per side, depending on the thickness of the fillets. Flip the salmon carefully using a spatula to avoid breaking it.
6. While the salmon is grilling, baste it with the remaining marinade occasionally to keep it moist and flavorful.
7. Remove the salmon from the grill once it is cooked through and flakes easily with a fork. Be careful not to overcook the salmon to keep it moist and tender.
8. Transfer the grilled salmon to a serving plate and garnish with fresh dill. Serve hot with lemon wedges on the side for an extra burst of citrus flavor.
9. Grilled salmon with lemon and dill pairs well with a variety of side dishes such as steamed vegetables, roasted potatoes, or a fresh salad. Enjoy this healthy and delicious meal packed with omega-3 fatty acids, protein, and refreshing flavors!

Note: Grilled salmon with lemon and dill is a simple yet flavorful dish that showcases the natural richness of the salmon. The combination of zesty lemon, aromatic dill, and perfectly grilled salmon creates a delicious and nutritious meal. This dish is not only satisfying to the taste buds but also provides essential nutrients like omega-3 fatty acids, which are beneficial for heart health and overall well-being. Enjoy this grilled salmon recipe as a wholesome main course for lunch or dinner, and savor the vibrant flavors that will leave you craving for more.

Quinoa and Vegetable Stir-Fry

Ingredients for Quinoa and Vegetable Stir-Fry:

- ✓ 1 cup quinoa
- ✓ 2 cups vegetable broth or water
- ✓ 2 tablespoons oil (such as olive oil or sesame oil)
- ✓ 2 cloves garlic, minced
- ✓ 1 onion, diced
- ✓ 1 carrot, diced
- ✓ 1 bell pepper, diced
- ✓ 1 zucchini, diced
- ✓ 1 cup broccoli florets
- ✓ 1 cup snap peas
- ✓ 2 tablespoons soy sauce or tamari (for gluten-free option)
- ✓ 1 tablespoon rice vinegar
- ✓ 1 teaspoon honey or maple syrup (optional)
- ✓ Salt and pepper, to taste
- ✓ Sesame seeds and chopped green onions for garnish (optional)

Instructions:

1. Rinse the quinoa thoroughly under cold water to remove any bitter coating. In a saucepan, combine the quinoa and vegetable broth (or water) and bring to a boil. Reduce the heat to low, cover, and simmer for about 15-20 minutes or until the quinoa is cooked and the liquid is absorbed. Remove from heat and let it sit covered for 5 minutes. Fluff with a fork.

2. In a large skillet or wok, heat the oil over medium heat. Add the minced garlic and diced onion, and sauté for 2-3 minutes until fragrant and lightly golden.

3. Add the diced carrot, bell pepper, zucchini, broccoli florets, and snap peas to the skillet. Stir-fry the vegetables for about 5-7 minutes or until they are tender-crisp.

4. In a small bowl, whisk together the soy sauce (or tamari), rice vinegar, and honey (or maple syrup) until well combined. Pour the sauce over the vegetables in the skillet and stir to coat evenly.

5. Add the cooked quinoa to the skillet and stir-fry for an additional 2-3 minutes, allowing the flavors to meld together.

6. Season with salt and pepper to taste. Adjust the seasoning or add more soy sauce if desired.

7. Remove from heat and garnish with sesame seeds and chopped green onions for extra flavor and presentation.

8. Serve the quinoa and vegetable stir-fry as a delicious and nutritious main course. It can also be enjoyed as a side dish or paired with protein of your choice such as tofu, chicken, or shrimp.

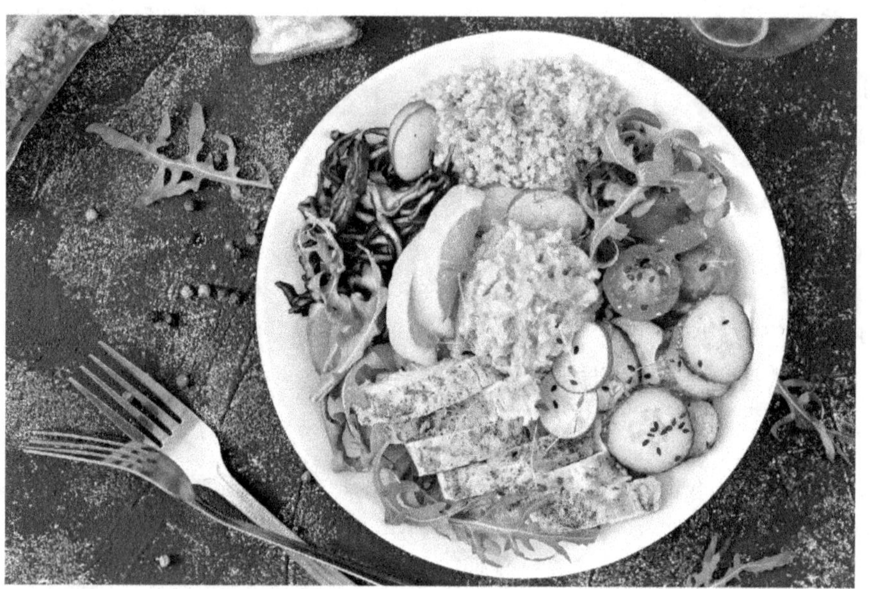

This quinoa and vegetable stir-fry is a versatile and satisfying dish that showcases the vibrant colors and textures of fresh vegetables. It provides a balanced combination of plant-based protein from quinoa and a variety of vitamins and minerals from the colorful vegetables. The stir-frying technique preserves the crispness and nutrients of the vegetables while infusing them with the savory flavors of garlic and soy sauce. This recipe is not only quick and easy to prepare but also a great way to incorporate wholesome ingredients into your meals. Enjoy this nutritious and delicious stir-fry as a healthy and filling option for lunch or dinner.

pinach and Mushroom Stuffed Chicken Breast

ngredients:

- ✓ 2 boneless, skinless chicken breasts
- ✓ 2 cups fresh spinach, chopped
- ✓ 1 cup mushrooms, sliced
- ✓ 1/2 cup shredded mozzarella cheese
- ✓ 2 cloves garlic, minced
- ✓ 1 tablespoon olive oil
- ✓ 1/2 teaspoon dried thyme
- ✓ Salt and pepper, to taste
- ✓ Toothpicks (optional)

nstructions:

1. Preheat your oven to 375°F (190°C).
2. Using a sharp knife, make a horizontal slit in the thickest part of each chicken breast to create a pocket. Be careful not to cut all the way through.
3. In a skillet, heat the olive oil over medium heat. Add the minced garlic and sauté for about 1 minute until fragrant.
4. Add the sliced mushrooms to the skillet and cook until they release their moisture and start to brown, about 5-6 minutes.
5. Add the chopped spinach to the skillet and cook for another 2-3 minutes until wilted. Remove from heat.
6. Stir in the shredded mozzarella cheese and dried thyme into the spinach and mushroom mixture. Season with salt and pepper to taste.
7. Stuff each chicken breast with the spinach and mushroom mixture, being careful not to overstuff. If needed, use toothpicks to secure the opening.
8. Heat a skillet over medium-high heat and add a drizzle of olive oil. Sear the stuffed chicken breasts for about 2-3 minutes on each side until browned.
9. Transfer the seared chicken breasts to a baking dish and place them in the preheated oven.
10. Bake for 20-25 minutes or until the chicken is cooked through and no longer pink in the center. The internal temperature should reach 165°F (75°C).
11. Remove from the oven and let the chicken rest for a few minutes before slicing.
12. Serve the spinach and mushroom stuffed chicken breasts as a delicious and satisfying main course. Pair it with a side of roasted vegetables, steamed rice, or a fresh salad for a complete meal.

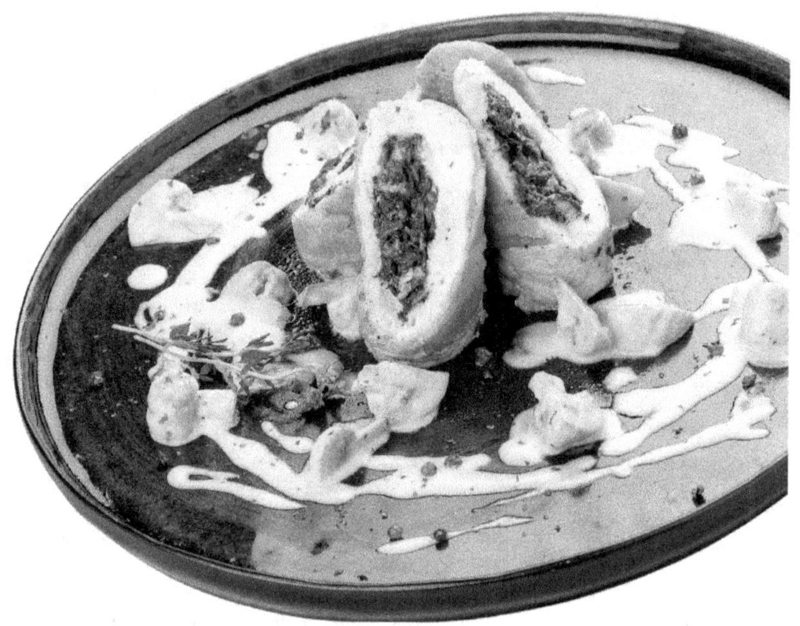

This recipe combines the lean protein of chicken breast with the earthy flavors of spinach and mushrooms. It's a wholesome and nutrient-rich dish that provides a good source of vitamins, minerals, and fiber. The melted mozzarella cheese adds a creamy and cheesy element to the filling, making every bite flavorful and satisfying. Whether you're looking for a quick and easy weeknight dinner or an impressive dish to serve to guests, this spinach and mushroom stuffed chicken breast is sure to please. Enjoy the combination of textures and flavors in this delicious and healthy recipe

entil and Vegetable Curry

gredients:

- ✓ 1 cup dried lentils
- ✓ 1 tablespoon olive oil
- ✓ 1 onion, chopped
- ✓ 3 cloves garlic, minced
- ✓ 1 tablespoon curry powder
- ✓ 1 teaspoon ground cumin
- ✓ 1 teaspoon ground turmeric
- ✓ 1 teaspoon paprika
- ✓ 1 can (14 ounces) diced tomatoes
- ✓ 1 can (14 ounces) coconut milk
- ✓ 2 cups mixed vegetables (such as carrots, bell peppers, peas)
- ✓ Salt and pepper, to taste
- ✓ Fresh cilantro, for garnish

structions:

1. Rinse the lentils under cold water and set aside.
2. In a large pot or Dutch oven, heat the olive oil over medium heat. Add the chopped onion and minced garlic, and sauté for about 5 minutes until the onion becomes translucent.
3. Add the curry powder, ground cumin, ground turmeric, and paprika to the pot. Stir well to coat the onions and garlic with the spices, and cook for another minute to release their flavors.
4. Add the diced tomatoes (with their juices) and coconut milk to the pot. Stir to combine.
5. Drain and rinse the lentils, then add them to the pot. Stir well to incorporate.
6. Bring the mixture to a boil, then reduce the heat to low and cover the pot. Let it simmer for about 20-25 minutes, or until the lentils are tender.
7. While the lentils are cooking, prepare your choice of mixed vegetables. You can chop carrots, bell peppers, and any other vegetables you prefer into bite-sized pieces.
8. Add the mixed vegetables to the pot and cook for an additional 10 minutes, or until the vegetables are cooked to your desired tenderness.
9. Season the lentil and vegetable curry with salt and pepper to taste.
10. Serve the curry hot, garnished with fresh cilantro. It pairs well with steamed rice or naan bread.

his lentil and vegetable curry is a hearty and nutritious dish that combines the protein-rich lentils with a ariety of colorful vegetables. The aromatic blend of spices adds depth and flavor to the curry, while the oconut milk provides a creamy and satisfying base. It's a versatile recipe that can be customized with your avorite vegetables and spice levels. Enjoy the comforting warmth and delicious flavors of this wholesome entil and vegetable curry, which is not only quick to make but also packed with essential nutrients and fiber.

Chapter 4: Side Dishes and Salads

Roasted Brussels Sprouts with Balsamic Glaze

Ingredients:

- ✓ 1 pound Brussels sprouts, trimmed and halved
- ✓ 2 tablespoons olive oil
- ✓ Salt and pepper, to taste
- ✓ 2 tablespoons balsamic vinegar
- ✓ 1 tablespoon honey or maple syrup (optional)
- ✓ Optional toppings: grated Parmesan cheese, chopped walnuts

Instructions:

1. Preheat your oven to 425°F (220°C).
2. In a large bowl, toss the Brussels sprouts with olive oil, salt, and pepper until they are well coated.
3. Arrange the Brussels sprouts in a single layer on a baking sheet.
4. Roast the Brussels sprouts in the preheated oven for about 20-25 minutes, or until they are tender and golden brown. Stir them once or twice during cooking to ensure even browning.
5. While the Brussels sprouts are roasting, prepare the balsamic glaze. In a small saucepan, combine the balsamic vinegar and honey or maple syrup (if using). Bring the mixture to a simmer over medium heat, stirring occasionally. Let it simmer for about 5 minutes until the glaze thickens slightly.
6. Remove the Brussels sprouts from the oven and transfer them to a serving dish.
7. Drizzle the balsamic glaze over the roasted Brussels sprouts.
8. Optional: Sprinkle grated Parmesan cheese and chopped walnuts on top for added flavor and texture.
9. Serve the roasted Brussels sprouts with balsamic glaze as a delicious and nutritious side dish or appetizer.

The roasting process brings out the natural sweetness and enhances the flavor of Brussels sprouts, while the balsamic glaze adds a tangy and slightly sweet element. This dish is a great way to enjoy the unique taste and texture of Brussels sprouts, and it pairs well with a variety of main courses. Whether you're serving it as a side dish for a family dinner or as an appetizer at a gathering, these roasted Brussels sprouts with balsamic glaze are sure to impress with their rich flavors and beautiful presentation.

Kale and Quinoa Salad

Ingredients:

- ✓ 1 cup cooked quinoa
- ✓ 2 cups kale leaves, chopped
- ✓ 1 cup cherry tomatoes, halved
- ✓ 1/2 cup cucumber, diced
- ✓ 1/4 cup red onion, thinly sliced
- ✓ 1/4 cup feta cheese, crumbled
- ✓ 2 tablespoons fresh lemon juice
- ✓ 2 tablespoons extra-virgin olive oil
- ✓ 1 garlic clove, minced
- ✓ Salt and pepper, to taste

Instructions:

1. In a large mixing bowl, combine the cooked quinoa, chopped kale, cherry tomatoes, cucumber, and red onion.

2. In a separate small bowl, whisk together the lemon juice, olive oil, minced garlic, salt, and pepper to make the dressing.

3. Pour the dressing over the quinoa and kale mixture and toss well to combine, ensuring that all ingredients are coated in the dressing.

4. Let the salad sit for at least 10 minutes to allow the flavors to meld together and the kale to soften slightly.

5. Just before serving, sprinkle the crumbled feta cheese over the salad and give it a final toss.

6. Taste and adjust the seasoning if needed.

7. Serve the kale and quinoa salad as a refreshing and nutritious side dish or as a light and satisfying main course.

This salad is packed with wholesome ingredients like quinoa, kale, and fresh vegetables, making it a great source of fiber, vitamins, and minerals. The lemony dressing adds a tangy and zesty flavor, while the feta cheese provides a creamy and salty element. Enjoy this vibrant and nourishing kale and quinoa salad as a delicious way to incorporate healthy ingredients into your diet.

Garlic and Herb Roasted Sweet Potatoes

Ingredients:

- ✓ 2 large sweet potatoes, peeled and cut into 1-inch cubes
- ✓ 3 tablespoons olive oil
- ✓ 4 cloves garlic, minced
- ✓ 1 teaspoon dried rosemary
- ✓ 1 teaspoon dried thyme
- ✓ 1/2 teaspoon salt
- ✓ 1/4 teaspoon black pepper

Instructions:

1. Preheat the oven to 425°F (220°C).

2. In a large mixing bowl, combine the sweet potato cubes, olive oil, minced garlic, dried rosemary, dried thyme, salt, and black pepper.

3. Toss the sweet potatoes until they are evenly coated with the oil and seasonings.

4. Spread the sweet potato cubes in a single layer on a baking sheet lined with parchment paper.

5. Place the baking sheet in the preheated oven and roast for about 25-30 minutes, or until the sweet potatoes are tender and golden brown, flipping them halfway through the cooking time for even browning.

6. Remove the roasted sweet potatoes from the oven and let them cool slightly before serving.

These garlic and herb roasted sweet potatoes make a delicious and nutritious side dish. The combination of garlic, rosemary, and thyme adds a savory and aromatic flavor to the sweet potatoes, enhancing their natural sweetness. Serve them alongside your favorite main course or enjoy them on their own as a tasty and satisfying snack.

Cucumber and Tomato Salad

Ingredients:

- ✓ 2 cucumbers, thinly sliced
- ✓ 2 tomatoes, diced
- ✓ 1/2 red onion, thinly sliced
- ✓ 1/4 cup fresh parsley, chopped
- ✓ 2 tablespoons olive oil
- ✓ 1 tablespoon lemon juice
- ✓ Salt and pepper to taste

Instructions:

1. In a large mixing bowl, combine the sliced cucumbers, diced tomatoes, thinly sliced red onion, and chopped parsley.

2. In a small bowl, whisk together the olive oil and lemon juice to make the dressing. Season with salt and pepper to taste.

3. Pour the dressing over the cucumber and tomato mixture and toss well to coat all the ingredients.

4. Let the salad sit for about 10 minutes to allow the flavors to meld together.

5. Give the salad a final toss before serving.

This refreshing cucumber and tomato salad is perfect for a light and healthy side dish. The crispness of the cucumbers, the juiciness of the tomatoes, and the tanginess of the dressing create a harmonious combination of flavors. It's a great addition to any summer meal or a refreshing option for picnics and gatherings. Enjoy the vibrant colors and fresh taste of this simple yet delicious salad.

Chapter 5: Soups and Stews

Immunity-Boosting Ginger Carrot Soup

Ingredients:

- ✓ 4 large carrots, peeled and chopped
- ✓ 1 onion, chopped
- ✓ 2 cloves of garlic, minced
- ✓ 1-inch piece of ginger, grated
- ✓ 4 cups vegetable broth
- ✓ 1 tablespoon olive oil
- ✓ 1 teaspoon turmeric powder
- ✓ 1/2 teaspoon cumin powder
- ✓ Salt and pepper to taste
- ✓ Fresh cilantro for garnish (optional)

Instructions:

1. Heat the olive oil in a large pot over medium heat. Add the chopped onions and minced garlic, and sauté until the onions are translucent.

2. Add the grated ginger, turmeric powder, and cumin powder to the pot, and cook for another minute, stirring well to coat the onions and garlic.

3. Add the chopped carrots to the pot and pour in the vegetable broth. Bring the mixture to a boil, then reduce the heat and simmer for about 15-20 minutes, or until the carrots are tender.

4. Remove the pot from heat and let it cool slightly. Using an immersion blender or regular blender, puree the soup until smooth and creamy.

5. Return the soup to the pot and place it back on the stove over low heat. Season with salt and pepper to taste, and simmer for a few more minutes to allow the flavors to meld together.

6. Ladle the ginger carrot soup into bowls and garnish with fresh cilantro if desired. Serve hot and enjoy the comforting and immune-boosting benefits of this nourishing soup.

Note: This ginger carrot soup is not only delicious but also packed with nutrients that can help support a healthy immune system. The ginger adds a zesty kick and has anti-inflammatory properties, while carrots provide beta-carotene and antioxidants. Enjoy this warm and soothing soup as a comforting meal or as part of your wellness routine.

Tomato and Basil Soup

Ingredients:

- ✓ 2 pounds ripe tomatoes, cored and chopped
- ✓ 1 onion, chopped
- ✓ 3 cloves of garlic, minced
- ✓ 2 tablespoons olive oil
- ✓ 4 cups vegetable broth
- ✓ 1/4 cup fresh basil leaves, chopped
- ✓ 1 teaspoon dried oregano
- ✓ Salt and pepper to taste
- ✓ Optional toppings: fresh basil leaves, grated Parmesan cheese, croutons

Instructions:

1. Heat the olive oil in a large pot over medium heat. Add the chopped onions and minced garlic, and sauté until the onions are translucent.

2. Add the chopped tomatoes to the pot and cook for about 5 minutes, stirring occasionally, until the tomatoes start to soften.

3. Pour in the vegetable broth and add the dried oregano. Bring the mixture to a boil, then reduce the heat and simmer for about 15-20 minutes, or until the tomatoes are completely tender.

4. Remove the pot from heat and let it cool slightly. Using an immersion blender or regular blender, puree the soup until smooth and creamy.

5. Return the soup to the pot and place it back on the stove over low heat. Stir in the chopped basil leaves and season with salt and pepper to taste. Simmer for a few more minutes to allow the flavors to meld together.

6. Ladle the tomato and basil soup into bowls. Serve hot and garnish with additional fresh basil leaves, grated Parmesan cheese, or croutons if desired. Enjoy the comforting flavors of this classic soup, perfect for any time of the year.

Hearty Vegetable and Bean Stew

Ingredients:

- ✓ 1 tablespoon olive oil
- ✓ 1 onion, diced
- ✓ 3 cloves of garlic, minced
- ✓ 2 carrots, peeled and chopped
- ✓ 2 celery stalks, chopped
- ✓ 1 bell pepper, diced
- ✓ 1 zucchini, chopped
- ✓ 1 can diced tomatoes
- ✓ 3 cups vegetable broth
- ✓ 1 can kidney beans, drained and rinsed
- ✓ 1 can chickpeas, drained and rinsed
- ✓ 1 teaspoon dried thyme
- ✓ 1 teaspoon paprika
- ✓ Salt and pepper to taste
- ✓ Fresh parsley, chopped (for garnish)

Instructions:

1. Heat the olive oil in a large pot over medium heat. Add the diced onion and minced garlic, and sauté until the onions are soft and fragrant.

2. Add the chopped carrots, celery, bell pepper, and zucchini to the pot. Cook for about 5 minutes, stirring occasionally, until the vegetables start to soften.

3. Pour in the diced tomatoes and vegetable broth. Add the drained kidney beans and chickpeas. Stir in the dried thyme and paprika. Season with salt and pepper to taste.

4. Bring the stew to a boil, then reduce the heat and simmer for about 20-25 minutes, or until the vegetables are tender.

5. Taste the stew and adjust the seasoning if needed. If you prefer a thicker consistency, you can use a potato masher or the back of a spoon to lightly mash some of the vegetables and beans.

6. Remove the pot from heat and let it sit for a few minutes to allow the flavors to meld together. Serve the hearty vegetable and bean stew hot, garnished with fresh parsley. Enjoy this comforting and nutritious meal on its own or with a side of crusty bread.

Coconut Curry Lentil Soup

Ingredients:

- ✓ 1 tablespoon coconut oil
- ✓ 1 onion, diced
- ✓ 3 cloves of garlic, minced
- ✓ 1 tablespoon grated ginger
- ✓ 2 carrots, peeled and chopped
- ✓ 1 bell pepper, diced
- ✓ 1 cup red lentils
- ✓ 1 can coconut milk
- ✓ 3 cups vegetable broth
- ✓ 2 teaspoons curry powder
- ✓ 1 teaspoon turmeric
- ✓ 1/2 teaspoon cumin
- ✓ Salt and pepper to taste
- ✓ Fresh cilantro, chopped (for garnish)
- ✓ Lime wedges (for serving)

Instructions:

1. Heat the coconut oil in a large pot over medium heat. Add the diced onion and cook until softened and translucent.

2. Add the minced garlic and grated ginger to the pot and sauté for another minute until fragrant.

3. Add the chopped carrots and bell pepper to the pot and cook for a few minutes until slightly softened.

4. Rinse the red lentils under cold water and add them to the pot. Stir to combine with the vegetables.

5. Pour in the coconut milk and vegetable broth. Add the curry powder, turmeric, and cumin. Season with salt and pepper to taste.

6. Bring the soup to a boil, then reduce the heat to low and simmer for about 20-25 minutes, or until the lentils are tender and cooked through.

7. Taste the soup and adjust the seasoning if needed. If you prefer a smoother consistency, you can use an immersion blender to blend a portion of the soup, or transfer a portion to a blender and blend until smooth before returning it to the pot.

8. Serve the coconut curry lentil soup hot, garnished with fresh cilantro and a squeeze of lime juice. Enjoy this flavorful and nourishing soup as a comforting meal on its own or with a side of naan bread or rice.

Chapter 6: Snacks and Appetizers

Turmeric-Spiced Roasted Chickpeas

Ingredients:

- ✓ 1 can chickpeas (15 ounces), rinsed and drained
- ✓ 1 tablespoon olive oil
- ✓ 1 teaspoon turmeric powder
- ✓ 1/2 teaspoon cumin powder
- ✓ 1/2 teaspoon paprika
- ✓ 1/4 teaspoon garlic powder
- ✓ 1/4 teaspoon salt
- ✓ 1/4 teaspoon black pepper

Instructions:

1. Preheat your oven to 400°F (200°C) and line a baking sheet with parchment paper.

2. In a bowl, combine the olive oil, turmeric powder, cumin powder, paprika, garlic powder, salt, and black pepper. Mix well to create a spice mixture.

3. Add the rinsed and drained chickpeas to the bowl with the spice mixture. Toss the chickpeas until they are well coated with the spices.

4. Spread the seasoned chickpeas in a single layer on the prepared baking sheet.

5. Roast the chickpeas in the preheated oven for about 25-30 minutes, or until they are crispy and golden brown. Make sure to shake the baking sheet halfway through to ensure even cooking.

6. Once the chickpeas are roasted to your desired crispiness, remove them from the oven and let them cool slightly before serving.

7. Serve the turmeric-spiced roasted chickpeas as a crunchy and flavorful snack on their own or as a topping for salads, soups, or grain bowls.

8. Store any leftovers in an airtight container at room temperature for up to a week. Enjoy the delicious and healthy snack whenever you need a tasty pick-me-up!

Guacamole with Fresh Veggies

Ingredients:

- ✓ 2 ripe avocados
- ✓ 1 small tomato, diced
- ✓ 1/4 cup red onion, finely chopped
- ✓ 1/4 cup cilantro, chopped
- ✓ 1 jalapeno pepper, seeded and finely chopped (optional, for heat)
- ✓ 1 lime, juiced
- ✓ 1 garlic clove, minced
- ✓ Salt and pepper to taste

For serving:

Assorted fresh vegetables such as sliced bell peppers, carrot sticks, celery sticks, cucumber slices, etc.

Instructions:

1. Cut the avocados in half and remove the pits. Scoop out the flesh into a bowl.

2. Use a fork to mash the avocados until desired consistency is reached (chunky or smooth).

3. Add the diced tomato, red onion, cilantro, jalapeno pepper (if using), lime juice, and minced garlic to the mashed avocados. Mix well to combine.

4. Season the guacamole with salt and pepper to taste. Adjust the lime juice and spices as desired.

5. Transfer the guacamole to a serving bowl and garnish with additional chopped cilantro, if desired.

6. Serve the guacamole with an assortment of fresh vegetables for dipping. Arrange the vegetable sticks around the guacamole bowl for a colorful presentation.

7. Enjoy the creamy and flavorful guacamole with the crispness of the fresh veggies. It makes a delicious and healthy appetizer or snack option for any occasion.

Smoked Salmon Cucumber Bites

Ingredients:

- ✓ 1 English cucumber
- ✓ 4 ounces of smoked salmon
- ✓ 4 tablespoons of cream cheese or Greek yogurt
- ✓ Fresh dill, chopped
- ✓ Lemon zest (optional)
- ✓ Salt and pepper to taste

Instructions:

1. Slice the cucumber into rounds, about 1/4 inch thick.

2. Arrange the cucumber rounds on a serving platter or plate.

3. Spread a thin layer of cream cheese or Greek yogurt on each cucumber round.

4. Cut the smoked salmon into small pieces that will fit on top of the cucumber rounds.

5. Place a piece of smoked salmon on each cucumber round, on top of the cream cheese or yogurt.

6. Sprinkle some fresh dill and a pinch of lemon zest (if desired) on top of each smoked salmon and cucumber bite.

7. Season with a pinch of salt and pepper.

8. Repeat the process with the remaining cucumber rounds and smoked salmon.

9. Serve the smoked salmon cucumber bites as a light and refreshing appetizer or snack option.

10. Enjoy the combination of cool cucumber, creamy cheese or yogurt, and flavorful smoked salmon in each bite.

weet Potato Fries with Greek Yogurt Dip

gredients:

r Sweet Potato Fries:

- ✓ 2 large sweet potatoes
- ✓ 2 tablespoons olive oil
- ✓ 1 teaspoon paprika
- ✓ 1/2 teaspoon garlic powder
- ✓ 1/2 teaspoon salt
- ✓ 1/4 teaspoon black pepper

or Greek Yogurt Dip:

- ✓ 1 cup Greek yogurt
- ✓ 1 tablespoon fresh lemon juice
- ✓ 1 tablespoon chopped fresh dill
- ✓ 1/2 teaspoon garlic powder
- ✓ Salt and pepper to taste

nstructions:

. Preheat the oven to 425°F (220°C) and line a baking sheet with parchment paper.

. Wash and peel the sweet potatoes. Cut them into long, thin strips resembling fries.

. In a large bowl, combine the sweet potato strips, olive oil, paprika, garlic powder, salt, and black pepper. oss until the sweet potatoes are evenly coated.

. Spread the sweet potato fries in a single layer on the prepared baking sheet.

. Bake in the preheated oven for about 25-30 minutes, flipping the fries halfway through, until they are crispy nd golden brown.

. While the fries are baking, prepare the Greek yogurt dip. In a small bowl, combine the Greek yogurt, lemon uice, chopped dill, garlic powder, salt, and pepper. Stir well to combine.

. Once the sweet potato fries are done, remove them from the oven and let them cool for a few minutes.

. Serve the sweet potato fries with the Greek yogurt dip on the side.

. Dip the crispy sweet potato fries into the creamy Greek yogurt dip for a delicious and healthier alternative to egular fries.

10. Enjoy the combination of the sweet and savory flavors and the creamy dip with each bite.

Chapter 7: Desserts and Treats

Dark Chocolate Avocado Mousse

Ingredients:

- ✓ 2 ripe avocados
- ✓ 1/4 cup unsweetened cocoa powder
- ✓ 1/4 cup maple syrup or honey
- ✓ 1/4 cup almond milk (or any milk of your choice)
- ✓ 1 teaspoon vanilla extract
- ✓ Pinch of salt
- ✓ Optional toppings: fresh berries, shaved chocolate, or chopped nuts

Instructions:

1. Cut the avocados in half and remove the pits. Scoop out the flesh and place it in a blender or food processor

2. Add the cocoa powder, maple syrup or honey, almond milk, vanilla extract, and a pinch of salt to the blender with the avocados.

3. Blend all the ingredients until smooth and creamy. You may need to stop and scrape down the sides of the blender a few times to ensure everything is well combined.

4. Taste the mousse and adjust the sweetness or cocoa powder according to your preference.

5. Once the mousse is smooth and well blended, transfer it to serving bowls or glasses.

6. Refrigerate the mousse for at least 30 minutes to allow it to set and chill.

7. Before serving, you can top the mousse with fresh berries, shaved chocolate, or chopped nuts for added texture and flavor.

8. Serve the dark chocolate avocado mousse chilled and enjoy its rich and creamy taste.

9. Indulge in this healthier dessert option that combines the goodness of avocados and dark chocolate.

10. Savor every spoonful of this decadent treat while knowing that you're nourishing your body with wholesome ingredients.

Berry Blast Smoothie Bowl

Ingredients:

- ✓ 1 cup frozen mixed berries (such as strawberries, blueberries, and raspberries)
- ✓ 1 ripe banana, sliced
- ✓ 1/2 cup unsweetened almond milk (or any milk of your choice)
- ✓ 1 tablespoon chia seeds
- ✓ 1 tablespoon honey or maple syrup (optional, for added sweetness)
- ✓ Toppings: fresh berries, sliced banana, granola, shredded coconut, chia seeds

Instructions:

1. In a blender, combine the frozen mixed berries, sliced banana, almond milk, chia seeds, and honey or maple syrup (if using).

2. Blend all the ingredients until smooth and creamy. If needed, you can add more almond milk to achieve your desired consistency.

3. Pour the berry blast smoothie into a bowl.

4. Top the smoothie bowl with fresh berries, sliced banana, granola, shredded coconut, and chia seeds. Feel free to add any other toppings of your choice.

5. Enjoy the smoothie bowl immediately with a spoon, savoring the combination of sweet and tangy flavors and the refreshing texture.

6. This berry blast smoothie bowl is not only delicious but also packed with antioxidants and nutrients from the mixed berries and chia seeds.

7. It's a perfect way to start your day or refuel after a workout, providing you with energy and nourishment.

8. Customize your smoothie bowl with different toppings and enjoy a nutritious and vibrant breakfast or snack.

9. Experiment with different combinations of fruits and toppings to create your own unique and flavorful smoothie bowls.

10. Indulge in this colorful and nutritious treat that will leave you feeling satisfied and refreshed.

Almond Butter Energy Balls

Ingredients:

- ✓ 1 cup rolled oats
- ✓ 1/2 cup almond butter
- ✓ 1/4 cup honey or maple syrup
- ✓ 1/4 cup ground flaxseed
- ✓ 1/4 cup shredded coconut
- ✓ 1/4 cup mini chocolate chips (optional)
- ✓ 1 teaspoon vanilla extract
- ✓ Pinch of salt

Instructions:

1. In a large mixing bowl, combine rolled oats, almond butter, honey or maple syrup, ground flaxseed, shredded coconut, mini chocolate chips (if using), vanilla extract, and a pinch of salt.

2. Stir all the ingredients together until well combined. If the mixture is too dry, you can add a little more almond butter or honey/maple syrup.

3. Once the mixture is well combined, use your hands to roll it into small balls, about 1 inch in diameter.

4. Place the almond butter energy balls on a baking sheet lined with parchment paper.

5. Refrigerate the energy balls for at least 30 minutes to allow them to firm up.

6. After refrigeration, the energy balls can be stored in an airtight container in the refrigerator for up to two weeks.

7. These almond butter energy balls are a perfect on-the-go snack, packed with protein, fiber, and healthy fats.

8. Enjoy them as a quick pick-me-up during the day or as a pre or post-workout snack to fuel your body.

9. Feel free to customize the energy balls by adding chopped nuts, dried fruits, or other mix-ins of your choice.

10. Indulge in these delicious and nutritious almond butter energy balls that will satisfy your cravings and provide you with a boost of energy.

Banana Ice Cream with Mixed Berries

Ingredients:

ripe bananas, frozen

cup mixed berries (such as strawberries, blueberries, raspberries)

/4 cup almond milk (or any other plant-based milk)

tablespoon honey or maple syrup (optional, for added sweetness)

teaspoon vanilla extract

Toppings of your choice (such as shredded coconut, chopped nuts, or additional fresh berries)

Instructions:

. Peel the ripe bananas and cut them into small slices. Place the banana slices in a freezer bag or container and freeze them for at least 4 hours or overnight.

2. Once the bananas are frozen, transfer them to a blender or food processor.

3. Add the mixed berries, almond milk, honey or maple syrup (if using), and vanilla extract to the blender.

4. Blend the mixture until smooth and creamy. You may need to stop and scrape down the sides of the blender or food processor a few times.

5. Once the mixture is well blended and resembles a soft-serve ice cream consistency, it is ready.

6. If you prefer a firmer texture, transfer the banana ice cream to a container and freeze it for an additional 1-2 hours.

7. Serve the banana ice cream in bowls or cones, and top it with your favorite toppings, such as shredded coconut, chopped nuts, or additional fresh berries.

8. Enjoy the creamy and refreshing banana ice cream with mixed berries as a healthier alternative to traditional ice cream.

9. This recipe is not only delicious but also packed with natural sweetness from the ripe bananas and antioxidants from the mixed berries.

10. Indulge in this guilt-free treat that will satisfy your sweet cravings while providing you with vitamins, minerals, and fiber from the fruits.

11. Feel free to experiment with different combinations of fruits and toppings to create your own variations of this delightful frozen dessert

30-DAY MEAL PLANNER

DAY 1

Date: _____________________   **CIRCLE ONE: Weekday   Weekend**

Breakfast	**Time of day: ....am/pm**
Food/Beverage Items	**Amount/Serving size**

Lunch	**Time of day:**	**am/pm**
Food/Beverage Items	**Amount/Serving size**	

Dinner	**Time of day:**	**am/pm**
Food/Beverage Items	**Amount/Serving size**	

Snacks

Time of day	Food/Beverage Items	Amount/Serving Size
________am/pm		
________am/pm		
________am/pm		

Estimated Daily Water Intake: _____________ounces/cups

DAY 2

Date: ___________________   **CIRCLE ONE:** Weekday   Weekend

Breakfast	**Time of day:** …………………….am/pm
Food/Beverage Items	**Amount/Serving size**

Lunch	**Time of day:** am/pm
Food/Beverage Items	**Amount/Serving size**

Dinner	**Time of day:** am/pm
Food/Beverage Items	**Amount/Serving size**

Snacks

Time of day	Food/Beverage Items	Amount/Serving Size
________am/pm		
________am/pm		
________am/pm		

Estimated Daily Water Intake: ______________ounces/cups

DAY 3

Date: _____________________   **CIRCLE ONE: Weekday   Weekend**

Breakfast	Time of day: ……………………..am/pm
Food/Beverage Items	**Amount/Serving size**

Lunch	Time of day: am/pm
Food/Beverage Items	**Amount/Serving size**

Dinner	Time of day: am/pm
Food/Beverage Items	**Amount/Serving size**

Snacks

Time of day	Food/Beverage Items	Amount/Serving Size
_________am/pm		
_________am/pm		
_________am/pm		

Estimated Daily Water Intake: _____________ounces/cups

DAY 4

Date: ______________________   **CIRCLE ONE: Weekday   Weekend**

Breakfast	**Time of day:** ....am/pm
Food/Beverage Items	**Amount/Serving size**

Lunch	**Time of day:** am/pm
Food/Beverage Items	**Amount/Serving size**

Dinner	**Time of day:** am/pm
Food/Beverage Items	**Amount/Serving size**

Snacks

Time of day	**Food/Beverage Items**	**Amount/Serving Size**
________am/pm		
________am/pm		
________am/pm		

Estimated Daily Water Intake: ____________ounces/cups

DAY 5

Date: _____________________   **CIRCLE ONE: Weekday   Weekend**

Breakfast	**Time of day: ……………………..am/pm**
Food/Beverage Items	**Amount/Serving size**

Lunch	**Time of day:** **am/pm**
Food/Beverage Items	**Amount/Serving size**

Dinner	**Time of day:** **am/pm**
Food/Beverage Items	**Amount/Serving size**

Snacks

Time of day	Food/Beverage Items	Amount/Serving Size
________am/pm		
________am/pm		
________am/pm		

Estimated Daily Water Intake: _____________ounces/cups

DAY 6

Date: _____________________   **CIRCLE ONE: Weekday   Weekend**

Breakfast	Time of day: ……………………..am/pm
Food/Beverage Items	**Amount/Serving size**

Lunch	Time of day: am/pm
Food/Beverage Items	**Amount/Serving size**

Dinner	Time of day: am/pm
Food/Beverage Items	**Amount/Serving size**

Snacks

Time of day	Food/Beverage Items	Amount/Serving Size
_________am/pm		
_________am/pm		
_________am/pm		

Estimated Daily Water Intake: _____________ounces/cups

DAY 7

Date: ___________________   **CIRCLE ONE: Weekday   Weekend**

Breakfast	Time of day: ....am/pm
Food/Beverage Items	**Amount/Serving size**

Lunch	Time of day: am/pm
Food/Beverage Items	**Amount/Serving size**

Dinner	Time of day: am/pm
Food/Beverage Items	**Amount/Serving size**

Snacks

Time of day	Food/Beverage Items	Amount/Serving Size
________am/pm		
________am/pm		
________am/pm		

Estimated Daily Water Intake: _____________ounces/cups

DAY 8

Date: ___________________   CIRCLE ONE: Weekday   Weekend

Breakfast	Time of day: ....am/pm
Food/Beverage Items	**Amount/Serving size**

Lunch	Time of day: _______ am/pm
Food/Beverage Items	**Amount/Serving size**

Dinner	Time of day: _______ am/pm
Food/Beverage Items	**Amount/Serving size**

Snacks

Time of day	Food/Beverage Items	Amount/Serving Size
_______am/pm		
_______am/pm		
_______am/pm		

Estimated Daily Water Intake: _______________ounces/cups

DAY 9

Date: ___________________   **CIRCLE ONE: Weekday   Weekend**

Breakfast	Time of day: ………………….am/pm
Food/Beverage Items	**Amount/Serving size**

Lunch	Time of day: am/pm
Food/Beverage Items	**Amount/Serving size**

Dinner	Time of day: am/pm
Food/Beverage Items	**Amount/Serving size**

Snacks

Time of day	Food/Beverage Items	Amount/Serving Size
_______am/pm		
_______am/pm		
_______am/pm		

Estimated Daily Water Intake: _____________ounces/cups

DAY 10

Date: ___________________   **CIRCLE ONE: Weekday   Weekend**

Breakfast	**Time of day:** …………………….am/pm
Food/Beverage Items	**Amount/Serving size**

Lunch	**Time of day:** am/pm
Food/Beverage Items	**Amount/Serving size**

Dinner	**Time of day:** am/pm
Food/Beverage Items	**Amount/Serving size**

Snacks

Time of day	**Food/Beverage Items**	**Amount/Serving Size**
_________am/pm		
_________am/pm		
_________am/pm		

Estimated Daily Water Intake: ______________ounces/cups

DAY 11

Date: ___________________   **CIRCLE ONE: Weekday   Weekend**

Breakfast	Time of day: ....am/pm
Food/Beverage Items	**Amount/Serving size**

Lunch	Time of day: am/pm
Food/Beverage Items	**Amount/Serving size**

Dinner	Time of day: am/pm
Food/Beverage Items	**Amount/Serving size**

Snacks

Time of day	Food/Beverage Items	Amount/Serving Size
_________am/pm		
_________am/pm		
_________am/pm		

Estimated Daily Water Intake: _____________ounces/cups

DAY 12

Date: _________________   **CIRCLE ONE: Weekday   Weekend**

Breakfast	Time of day: ……………………..am/pm
Food/Beverage Items	**Amount/Serving size**

Lunch	Time of day: am/pm
Food/Beverage Items	**Amount/Serving size**

Dinner	Time of day: am/pm
Food/Beverage Items	**Amount/Serving size**

Snacks

Time of day	Food/Beverage Items	Amount/Serving Size
_________am/pm		
_________am/pm		
_________am/pm		

Estimated Daily Water Intake: _____________ounces/cups

DAY 13

Date: _______________________   **CIRCLE ONE: Weekday   Weekend**

Breakfast	**Time of day: …………………….am/pm**
Food/Beverage Items	**Amount/Serving size**

Lunch	**Time of day: am/pm**
Food/Beverage Items	**Amount/Serving size**

Dinner	**Time of day: am/pm**
Food/Beverage Items	**Amount/Serving size**

Snacks

Time of day	Food/Beverage Items	Amount/Serving Size
________am/pm		
________am/pm		
________am/pm		

Estimated Daily Water Intake: _____________ounces/cups

DAY 14

Date: _____________________   **CIRCLE ONE: Weekday   Weekend**

Breakfast	**Time of day: ……………………am/pm**
Food/Beverage Items	**Amount/Serving size**

Lunch	**Time of day:**	**am/pm**
Food/Beverage Items	**Amount/Serving size**	

Dinner	**Time of day:**	**am/pm**
Food/Beverage Items	**Amount/Serving size**	

Snacks

Time of day	Food/Beverage Items	Amount/Serving Size
________am/pm		
________am/pm		
________am/pm		

Estimated Daily Water Intake: _____________ounces/cups

DAY 15

Date: _________________   **CIRCLE ONE: Weekday   Weekend**

Breakfast	**Time of day: ………………….am/pm**
Food/Beverage Items	**Amount/Serving size**

Lunch	**Time of day: am/pm**
Food/Beverage Items	**Amount/Serving size**

Dinner	**Time of day: am/pm**
Food/Beverage Items	**Amount/Serving size**

Snacks

Time of day	**Food/Beverage Items**	**Amount/Serving Size**
_________am/pm		
_________am/pm		
_________am/pm		

Estimated Daily Water Intake: _____________ounces/cups

DAY 16

Date: _____________________   **CIRCLE ONE: Weekday   Weekend**

Breakfast	**Time of day:** ………………………am/pm
Food/Beverage Items	**Amount/Serving size**

Lunch	**Time of day:** am/pm
Food/Beverage Items	**Amount/Serving size**

Dinner	**Time of day:** am/pm
Food/Beverage Items	**Amount/Serving size**

Snacks

Time of day	Food/Beverage Items	Amount/Serving Size
_________am/pm		
_________am/pm		
_________am/pm		

Estimated Daily Water Intake: _____________ounces/cups

DAY 17

Date: ___________________   **CIRCLE ONE: Weekday   Weekend**

Breakfast	**Time of day: …………………….am/pm**
Food/Beverage Items	**Amount/Serving size**

Lunch	**Time of day: am/pm**
Food/Beverage Items	**Amount/Serving size**

Dinner	**Time of day: am/pm**
Food/Beverage Items	**Amount/Serving size**

Snacks

Time of day	**Food/Beverage Items**	**Amount/Serving Size**
_______am/pm		
_______am/pm		
_______am/pm		

Estimated Daily Water Intake: _____________ounces/cups

DAY 18

Date: _____________________   **CIRCLE ONE: Weekday   Weekend**

Breakfast	Time of day: …………………….am/pm
Food/Beverage Items	**Amount/Serving size**

Lunch	Time of day: am/pm
Food/Beverage Items	**Amount/Serving size**

Dinner	Time of day: am/pm
Food/Beverage Items	**Amount/Serving size**

Snacks

Time of day	Food/Beverage Items	Amount/Serving Size
_________am/pm		
_________am/pm		
_________am/pm		

Estimated Daily Water Intake: _____________ounces/cups

DAY 19

Date: _____________________   **CIRCLE ONE: Weekday   Weekend**

Breakfast	Time of day: …………………….am/pm
Food/Beverage Items	**Amount/Serving size**

Lunch	Time of day: am/pm
Food/Beverage Items	**Amount/Serving size**

Dinner	Time of day: am/pm
Food/Beverage Items	**Amount/Serving size**

Snacks

Time of day	Food/Beverage Items	Amount/Serving Size
_________am/pm		
_________am/pm		
_________am/pm		

Estimated Daily Water Intake: _____________ounces/cups

DAY 20

Date: _________________   CIRCLE ONE: Weekday   Weekend

Breakfast	Time of day: …………………….am/pm
Food/Beverage Items	**Amount/Serving size**

Lunch	Time of day: ______ am/pm
Food/Beverage Items	**Amount/Serving size**

Dinner	Time of day: ______ am/pm
Food/Beverage Items	**Amount/Serving size**

Snacks

Time of day	Food/Beverage Items	Amount/Serving Size
________am/pm		
________am/pm		
________am/pm		

Estimated Daily Water Intake: ______________ounces/cups

DAY 21

Date: _____________________   **CIRCLE ONE: Weekday   Weekend**

Breakfast	Time of day: ………………….am/pm
Food/Beverage Items	**Amount/Serving size**

Lunch	Time of day: am/pm
Food/Beverage Items	**Amount/Serving size**

Dinner	Time of day: am/pm
Food/Beverage Items	**Amount/Serving size**

Snacks

Time of day	Food/Beverage Items	Amount/Serving Size
_______am/pm		
_______am/pm		
_______am/pm		

Estimated Daily Water Intake: _____________ounces/cups

DAY 22

Date: ___________________   **CIRCLE ONE: Weekday   Weekend**

Breakfast	**Time of day:** ....am/pm
Food/Beverage Items	**Amount/Serving size**

Lunch	**Time of day:** am/pm
Food/Beverage Items	**Amount/Serving size**

Dinner	**Time of day:** am/pm
Food/Beverage Items	**Amount/Serving size**

Snacks

Time of day	Food/Beverage Items	Amount/Serving Size
________am/pm		
________am/pm		
________am/pm		

Estimated Daily Water Intake: ______________ounces/cups

DAY 23

Date: _____________________   **CIRCLE ONE: Weekday   Weekend**

Breakfast	**Time of day: …………………….am/pm**
Food/Beverage Items	**Amount/Serving size**

Lunch	**Time of day:** **am/pm**
Food/Beverage Items	**Amount/Serving size**

Dinner	**Time of day:** **am/pm**
Food/Beverage Items	**Amount/Serving size**

Snacks

Time of day	**Food/Beverage Items**	**Amount/Serving Size**
_______am/pm		
_______am/pm		
_______am/pm		

Estimated Daily Water Intake: _____________ounces/cups

DAY 24

Date: _________________   **CIRCLE ONE: Weekday   Weekend**

Breakfast	**Time of day: …………………….am/pm**
Food/Beverage Items	**Amount/Serving size**

Lunch	**Time of day:**	**am/pm**
Food/Beverage Items	**Amount/Serving size**	

Dinner	**Time of day:**	**am/pm**
Food/Beverage Items	**Amount/Serving size**	

Snacks

Time of day	**Food/Beverage Items**	**Amount/Serving Size**
_________am/pm		
_________am/pm		
_________am/pm		

Estimated Daily Water Intake: _____________ounces/cups

DAY 25

Date: _____________________   **CIRCLE ONE: Weekday   Weekend**

Breakfast	Time of day: ………………….am/pm
Food/Beverage Items	**Amount/Serving size**

Lunch	Time of day: am/pm
Food/Beverage Items	**Amount/Serving size**

Dinner	Time of day: am/pm
Food/Beverage Items	**Amount/Serving size**

Snacks

Time of day	Food/Beverage Items	Amount/Serving Size
_________am/pm		
_________am/pm		
_________am/pm		

Estimated Daily Water Intake: _____________ounces/cups

DAY 26

Date: ___________________   **CIRCLE ONE: Weekday   Weekend**

Breakfast	Time of day: ....am/pm
Food/Beverage Items	**Amount/Serving size**

Lunch	Time of day: am/pm
Food/Beverage Items	**Amount/Serving size**

Dinner	Time of day: am/pm
Food/Beverage Items	**Amount/Serving size**

Snacks

Time of day	Food/Beverage Items	Amount/Serving Size
_______am/pm		
_______am/pm		
_______am/pm		

Estimated Daily Water Intake: _____________ounces/cups

DAY 27

Date: _________________   **CIRCLE ONE: Weekday   Weekend**

Breakfast	**Time of day: ....am/pm**
Food/Beverage Items	**Amount/Serving size**

Lunch	**Time of day: am/pm**
Food/Beverage Items	**Amount/Serving size**

Dinner	**Time of day: am/pm**
Food/Beverage Items	**Amount/Serving size**

Snacks

Time of day	Food/Beverage Items	Amount/Serving Size
_________am/pm		
_________am/pm		
_________am/pm		

Estimated Daily Water Intake: _____________ounces/cups

DAY 28

Date: _______________________   **CIRCLE ONE: Weekday   Weekend**

Breakfast	Time of day: ………………….am/pm
Food/Beverage Items	**Amount/Serving size**

Lunch	Time of day: am/pm
Food/Beverage Items	**Amount/Serving size**

Dinner	Time of day: am/pm
Food/Beverage Items	**Amount/Serving size**

Snacks

Time of day	Food/Beverage Items	Amount/Serving Size
_______am/pm		
_______am/pm		
_______am/pm		

Estimated Daily Water Intake: _____________ounces/cups

DAY 29

Date: ___________________   **CIRCLE ONE: Weekday   Weekend**

Breakfast	**Time of day:** ....am/pm
Food/Beverage Items	**Amount/Serving size**

Lunch	**Time of day:** am/pm
Food/Beverage Items	**Amount/Serving size**

Dinner	**Time of day:** am/pm
Food/Beverage Items	**Amount/Serving size**

Snacks

Time of day	Food/Beverage Items	Amount/Serving Size
________am/pm		
________am/pm		
________am/pm		

Estimated Daily Water Intake: _____________ounces/cups

DAY 30

Date: ___________________   **CIRCLE ONE: Weekday   Weekend**

Breakfast	**Time of day: ....am/pm**
Food/Beverage Items	**Amount/Serving size**

Lunch	**Time of day: am/pm**
Food/Beverage Items	**Amount/Serving size**

Dinner	**Time of day: am/pm**
Food/Beverage Items	**Amount/Serving size**

Snacks

Time of day	**Food/Beverage Items**	**Amount/Serving Size**
_________am/pm		
_________am/pm		
_________am/pm		

Estimated Daily Water Intake: _____________ounces/cups